Amantadine in Parkinson's Disease
An Expert Opinion

DISCLAIMER

Medicine is ever-changing science. As new research and clinical experience broaden our knowledge, changes in treatment and drug therapy are required. The authors and the publishers of this work have checked with sources believed to be reliable in their efforts to provide information that is complete and generally in accord with the standards accepted at the time of publication. However, in view of the possibility of human error or changes in medical sciences, neither the author nor the publisher nor any other party who has been involved in the preparation or publication of this work warrants that the information contained herein is in every respect accurate or complete, and they disclaim all responsibility for any errors or omissions or for the results obtained from use of information contained in this work. Readers are encourage to confirm the information contained herein with other sources. For example and in particular, readers are advised to check product information sheet included in the package of each medication they plan to administer to be certain that the information contained in this work is accurate and that changes have not been made in the recommended dose or in the contraindication for administration. This recommendation is of particular importance in connection with new or infrequently used medicine.

Amantadine in Parkinson's Disease
An Expert Opinion

Vinay Goyal
MD DM (AIIMS) FIAN
Ex-Professor of Neurology
All India Institute of Medical Sciences
New Delhi, India
Director Neurology
Medanta - The Medicity
Gurugram, Haryana, India

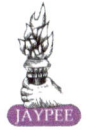

JAYPEE BROTHERS MEDICAL PUBLISHERS
The Health Sciences Publisher
New Delhi | London

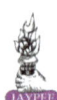 **Jaypee Brothers Medical Publishers (P) Ltd**

Headquarters
EMCA House
23/23-B, Ansari Road, Daryaganj
New Delhi 110 002, India
Landline: +91-11-23272143, +91-11-23272703
+91-11-23282021, +91-11-23245672
E-mail: jaypee@jaypeebrothers.com

Corporate Office
Jaypee Brothers Medical Publishers (P) Ltd.
4838/24, Ansari Road, Daryaganj
New Delhi 110 002, India
Phone: +91-11-43574357
Fax: +91-11-43574314
E-mail: jaypee@jaypeebrothers.com

Overseas Office
JP Medical Ltd.
83, Victoria Street, London
SW1H 0HW (UK)
Phone: +44-20 3170 8910
Fax: +44(0)20 3008 6180
E-mail: info@jpmedpub.com

Website: www.jaypeebrothers.com
Website: www.jaypeedigital.com

© 2022, Jaypee Brothers Medical Publishers

The views and opinions expressed in this book are solely those of the original contributor(s)/author(s) and do not necessarily represent those of editor(s) of the book.

All rights reserved by the author. No part of this publication may be reproduced, stored or transmitted in any form or by any means, electronic, mechanical, photocopying, recording or otherwise, without the prior permission in writing of the publishers.

All brand names and product names used in this book are trade names, service marks, trademarks or registered trademarks of their respective owners. The publisher is not associated with any product or vendor mentioned in this book.

Medical knowledge and practice change constantly. This book is designed to provide accurate, authoritative information about the subject matter in question. However, readers are advised to check the most current information available on procedures included and check information from the manufacturer of each product to be administered, to verify the recommended dose, formula, method and duration of administration, adverse effects and contraindications. It is the responsibility of the practitioner to take all appropriate safety precautions. Neither the publisher nor the author(s)/editor(s) assume any liability for any injury and/or damage to persons or property arising from or related to use of material in this book.

This book is sold on the understanding that the publisher is not engaged in providing professional medical services. If such advice or services are required, the services of a competent medical professional should be sought.

Every effort has been made where necessary to contact holders of copyright to obtain permission to reproduce copyright material. If any have been inadvertently overlooked, the publisher will be pleased to make the necessary arrangements at the first opportunity. The **CD/DVD-ROM** (if any) provided in the sealed envelope with this book is complimentary and free of cost. **It is Not meant for sale**.

Inquiries for bulk sales may be solicited at: jaypee@jaypeebrothers.com

Amantadine in Parkinson's Disease: An Expert Opinion **/ Vinay Goyal**

First Edition: **2022**

ISBN: 978-93-90595-61-7

Preface

Parkinson's disease is a common neurodegenerative disease affecting the elderly population. The disease remains a huge challenge and its prevalence is expected to double worldwide by 2040.

It is important to distinguish it from other neurodegenerative diseases; therefore, understanding its symptoms is important which can aid in better diagnosis as well as more specific management. The management of Parkinson's disease can often be challenging; hence, it is important to increase awareness of other therapeutic options. Levodopa is the mainstay in the pharmacological management of Parkinson's disease; however, the drug has been associated with some side effects. Additionally, it is important that treatment is individualized and tailored for individual patients based on their condition.

Amantadine has been in use since 1966; however, its use in Parkinson's disease initiated in 1968, when an old woman experienced a remarkable remission in her symptoms of rigidity, tremor, and akinesia. Since then, the drug has been utilized in the management of Parkinson's disease.

The book provides a comprehensive understanding on amantadine and its pharmacological and clinical efficacy.

Vinay Goyal

Contributors

Editor in Chief

Vinay Goyal MD DM (AIIMS) FIAN
Ex-Professor of Neurology
All India Institute of Medical Sciences
New Delhi, India
Director Neurology
Medanta - The Medicity
Gurugram, Haryana, India

Contributing Authors

Anup Kumar Thacker MD DNB DM MNAMS
Director, Division of Neurology
Medanta – The Medcity
Gurugram, Haryana, India

Chandrashekhar Agrawal MBBS MD DM
Senior Consultant
Department of Neurology
Sir Ganga Ram Hospital
New Delhi, India

Hrishikesh Kumar MD DM
Head, Department of Neurology
Director of Research
In Charge, Parkinson's Disease and Movement Disorders Program
Institute of Neurosciences
Kolkata, West Bengal, India

Pahari Ghosh MBBS MD MRCP FCCP DM FRCP
Senior Consultant Neurologist
Calcutta Medical Research Institute, Kolkata, India
B P Poddar Hospital, Kolkata, India
Belle Vue Clinic, Kolkata, India
Woodlands Hospital and Research Institute, Kolkata, India
Sri Aurobindo Seva Kendra, Kolkata, India

Rahul Kulkarni MD DM DNB FAAN
Consultant Neurologist
Deenanath Mangeshkar Hospital and Research Center
Pune, Maharashtra, India

SK Jaiswal MD DM
Consultant Neurologist
KIMS Hospital
Kondapur, Hyderabad, India

Sudhir V Shah MBBS MD DM
Consultant Neurologist
Neurology Centre
206-6-8 Sangini Complex
Near Parimal Crossing
Ellisbridge
Ahmedabad, Gujarat, India

Contents

1. Clinical Signs and Symptoms of Parkinson's Disease — **1**
Introduction 1
Epidemiology of Parkinson's Disease 1
Risk Factors of Parkinson'S Disease 3
Symptoms 3
Advanced Parkinson's Disease 7
Summary 8

2. Parkinson's Disease: Pathophysiology and Diagnosis — **10**
Pathophysiology 10
Diagnosis of Parkinson's Disease 11
Management of Parkinson's Disease 15
Summary 17

3. Role of Amantadine in Parkinson's Disease — **19**
Introduction and Basic Chemistry 19
Pharmacodynamic 19
Mechanism of Action of Amantadine 20
Clinical Indications 22
Pharmacokinetic Properties 23
Summary 26

4. Clinical Efficacy and Safety of Amantadine — **28**
Efficacy of Amantadine in Levodopa-induced Dyskinesia
in Parkinson's Disease 28
Postural Reflex Impairment In Parkinson's Disease 31
Efficacy of Amantadine In Freezing of Gait 31
Duration of Amantadine Benefit on Dyskinesia of
Severe Parkinson's Disease 33
Amantadine Effectiveness in Multiple System Atrophy and
Progressive Supranuclear Palsy 34
Use of Amantadine in Other Disorders 37
Summary 39

5. Amantadine: Dosage, Adverse Effects, and Drug–Drug Interactions 42

Dosage and Administration 42
Overdosage of Amantadine 43
Adverse Effects 44
Monitoring 46
Contraindications 46
Drug–Drug Interactions 47
Summary 47

Index 49

CHAPTER 1

Clinical Signs and Symptoms of Parkinson's Disease

INTRODUCTION

Parkinson's disease (PD) is the common neurodegenerative movement disorder.[1] The disease is characterized by the degeneration of dopaminergic (DA) neurons of the brain.[2] The disease is associated with motor symptoms and nonmotor symptoms.[3]

EPIDEMIOLOGY OF PARKINSON'S DISEASE

Globally, the prevalence of PD is estimated to be 10 million people and 1% of those above 60 years are affected with PD (see **Fig. 1**).[4] It is expected to double worldwide by 2040.[5]

With increase in age, the incidence and prevalence of PD increase. In some patients, the onset of PD is seen as early as 40 years and it accounts for 15–25% of all PD cases. In India, there is no homogeneous and large epidemiological data on PD. However, the prevalence rate over the age of 60 years was 247/100,000. Crude prevalence rate of 14.1 per 100,000 from rural Kashmir, 27/100,000 from Bengaluru, 16.1/100,000 from rural Bengal, and 328.3/100,000 in Mumbai (see **Fig. 2**).[6]

Clinical Signs and Symptoms of Parkinson's Disease

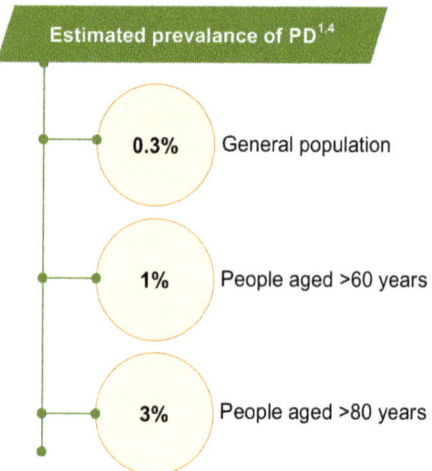

FIG. 1: Estimated prevalence of PD.

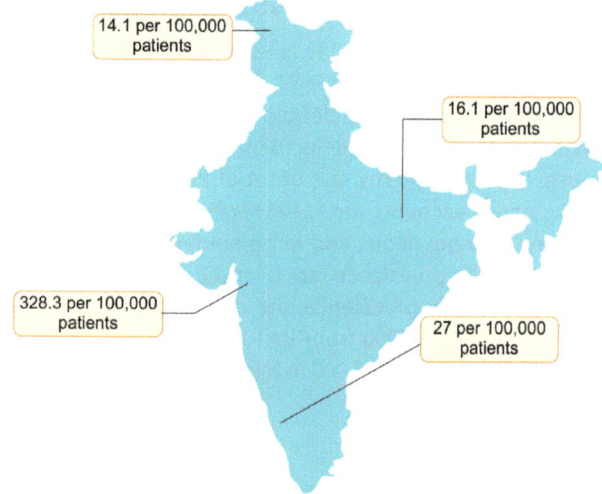

FIG. 2: Incidence and prevalence of PD-Indian context.

RISK FACTORS OF PARKINSON'S DISEASE

Various risk factors contribute toward PD, some of which include:[4,6]

- Age—most important risk factor
- Male—confers a moderate risk
- Family history
- *Environmental factors*: Pesticides and rural living
- Exposure to toxic levels of manganese, trichloroethylene, and carbon monoxide
- β2-adrenoreceptor antagonists
- Elevated cholesterol
- Head trauma, e.g., boxing
- High caloric intake
- Increased body mass index
- Inflammation associated with activation of microglia
- Oxidative stress
- Postinfection states

SYMPTOMS

The symptoms are given in **Figure 3**.

Motor Symptoms (Flowchart 1)

The important symptoms of PD include bradykinesia, tremor, rigidity, and postural instability.[3]

Bradykinesia

Bradykinesia is cardinal and earliest signs of Parkinsonism, which is the result of reduced dopamine levels in the brain. The term bradykinesia in Greek means slow movement, which is experienced by nearly 98% of people with PD. Bradykinesia can affect one limb, one side of your body, or your whole body, which can make you unnaturally still. Akinesia and hypokinesia

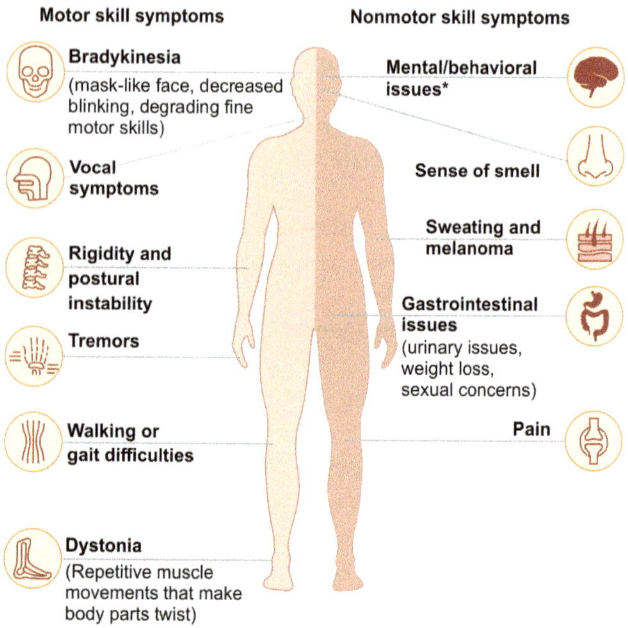

4 Clinical Signs and Symptoms of Parkinson's Disease

Motor skill symptoms
- **Bradykinesia** (mask-like face, decreased blinking, degrading fine motor skills)
- **Vocal symptoms**
- **Rigidity and postural instability**
- **Tremors**
- **Walking or gait difficulties**
- **Dystonia** (Repetitive muscle movements that make body parts twist)

Nonmotor skill symptoms
- **Mental/behavioral issues***
- **Sense of smell**
- **Sweating and melanoma**
- **Gastrointestinal issues** (urinary issues, weight loss, sexual concerns)
- **Pain**

*Include depression, anxiety, fatigue, sleep problems, and cognitive ability and personality changes.

FIG. 3: PD symptoms.

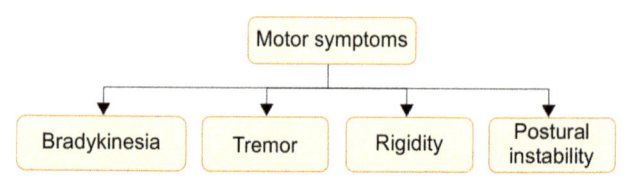

FLOWCHART 1: Motor symptoms observed in PD patients.

are terms, which are often used in relation to bradykinesia. Associated features are small handwriting (micrographia) or soft voice (hypophonia).[7]

Tremor

Another common symptom associated with PD is tremor. Tremor is defined as an involuntary, rhythmic movement that affects a part of the body, for example, hand, which is because of rapid and alternating contraction of agonistic and antagonistic muscles. Nearly, 70% of people with PD have a tremor at the time of diagnosis. Rest tremor is classic for PD. Rest tremor usually affects upper limbs, but legs, lips, and tongue may also be involved.[7]

Rigidity

One of another main motor symptoms of PD is rigidity, which is present in 90–99% of people. This leads to muscle aches, stiffness, or muscle fatigue.[7]

Postural Instability

Postural instability is one of late features of PD.[8,9] Within 2 years of PD diagnosis, nearly 34% of patients develop postural instability, which increases to 71% in 10 years and 92% at 15 years.[8]

Nonmotor Symptoms (Flowchart 2)

The nonmotor symptoms of PD include olfactory dysfunction, cognitive impairment, sleep disorder, pain, depression, anxiety, autonomic nervous dysfunction, etc., which can occur during PD or earlier than motor symptoms, adversely affecting the quality of life.[3]

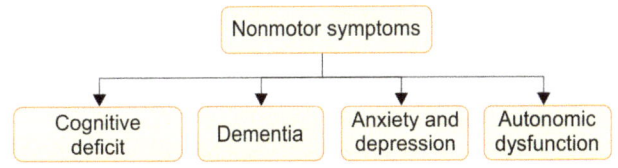

FLOWCHART 2: Nonmotor symptoms observed in PD patients.

6 Clinical Signs and Symptoms of Parkinson's Disease

Nonmotor symptoms are critical to diagnose as well as treat PD, as it has a significant impact on individual's quality of life, especially in case of advanced PD.[10] The nonmotor symptoms include cognitive impairment, neuropsychiatric symptoms, sleep disorders, and olfactory dysfunction. Some of these symptoms may precede motor symptoms in PD as early as 10 years. Compared with motor symptoms, the nonmotor symptoms have greater impact on quality of life and are significantly associated with reduced individual well-being. In patients with advanced PD, nonmotor symptoms play an important role in loss of independence. A survey evaluating the nonmotor symptoms of PD reported including sleep problems (84%), cognitive symptoms (76%), anxiety (65%), depression (56%), hallucinations (40%), and delusions (23%).[11]

It is difficult to put all nonmotor symptoms into one category and, therefore, following classification is recommended:[12]

- *Related to the disease process or pathophysiology*:
  - Dopaminergic origin
  - Nondopaminergic origin
- Related to a partial nonmotor origin (usually brainstem autonomic impairment with motor end result such as constipation or diplopia)
- Related to nonmotor fluctuations (cognitive, autonomic, and sensory subtypes)
  - Fluctuating
  - Constant
- *Related to PD drug therapy*:
  - Specific symptoms (e.g., hallucinations, delirium)
  - Syndromes—impulse control disorders, dopamine agonist withdrawal syndrome, Parkinson's hyperpyrexia syndrome (thermoregulatory failure and delirium)
- *Possibly genetically determined*:
  - Dementia in cases with glucocerebrosidase mutation
  - Depression and sleep disorders in cases with leucine-rich repeat kinase-2 mutation

- *Some symptoms may overlap*: For instance, hallucination as part of the advancing disease or nonmotor fluctuations in PD

In premotor stage of PD, some of the reported nonmotor symptoms have been shown in **Table 1**.[12]

ADVANCED PARKINSON'S DISEASE

Advanced PD is defined as onset of disabling motor symptoms.[13] The time span for a patient to reach advanced stage may reach usually in 5–10 years from the time of diagnosis. Dyskinesia and motor fluctuations are the most frequent motor symptoms in

TABLE 1: Nonmotor symptoms in the premotor Parkinson's disease (PD).	
Commonly associated—with reasonable evidence base	
Hyposmia (usually of late onset and idiopathic)	10 times increase in risk of developing PD + abnormal DAT scan—43% develop motor PD in 4 years
Rapid eye movement sleep behavior disorder	25–40% risk of developing a synucleinopathy at 5 years and 40–65% risk of developing a synucleinopathy at 10 years
Constipation	2.7–4.5 times increased risk of PD
Depression	2.4 times increased risk of developing PD
Described associations	
Excessive daytime sleepiness	3.3 times increased risk of PD
Fatigue (a sense of exhaustion as opposed to sleepiness)	In 45%—a premotor symptom
Pain (often unilateral and in affected limb)	34% increased risk of PD
Erectile dysfunction	3.8 times increased risk of PD

advanced PD. Meta-analyses have estimated 40% probability of developing dyskinesia and motor functions after 4 years of levodopa treatment. Motor fluctuations could get complex with progression of the disease.[13]

Parkinson's disease is considered advanced, if the patient experiences a fluctuating clinical state with alternating periods of good and poor symptom control. These fluctuations may affect both motor and NMS and they cannot be controlled using conventional therapy. Advanced PD gives rise to motor symptoms that respond poorly or not at all to oral levodopa. Symptoms include gait disorders, postural disorders, lack of stability, dysphagia, and dysarthria and they cause severe disability. Appearance of nonmotor complications and the development of disabling NMS (such as dementia, autonomic symptoms, pain, or psychiatric symptoms) are typical in patients with advanced PD.[13]

The timeline for progression to advanced PD varies from patient to patient. Various risk factors for advance PD include age, gender, disease duration, motor phenotype, olfactory changes, sleep behavior disorder, hallucinations, psychosis, and cognitive decline.[13]

SUMMARY

- Parkinson's disease is a common neurodegenerative movement disorder.
- Disease is characterized by the degeneration of DA neurons of the brain.
- The important motor symptoms of PD include tremor, rigidity, bradykinesia, and postural instability.
- Nonmotor symptoms include olfactory dysfunction, cognitive impairment, sleep disorder, pain, depression, anxiety, and autonomic nervous dysfunction.

REFERENCES

1. Balestrino R, Schapira AHV. Parkinson disease. Eur J Neurol. 2020;27(1):27-42.
2. Alieva AK, Filatova EV, Karabanov AV, Illarioshkin SN, Slominsky PA, Shadrina MI. Potential Biomarkers of the Earliest Clinical Stages of Parkinson's Disease. Parkinson's Dis. 2015;2015:294396.
3. Fathima ST, Fatima T, Mridula KR, Kumar KV, Rupam B. Association of brain-derived neurotrophic factor (Val66Met) polymorphism with the risk of Parkinson's disease and influence on clinical outcome. Indian J Biochem Biophys. 2020;57(4):192-201.
4. Pradahan M, Srivastava R. Etiology. Epidemiology, Diagnosis and Current Therapeutic Protocols for Parkinson's Disease (PD): An Overview. Med Surg Radiol. 2020;5(1):A186-91.
5. McFarthing K, Buff S, Rafaloff G, Dominey T, Wyse RK, Stott SRW. Parkinson's Disease Drug Therapies in the Clinical Trial Pipeline: 2020. J Parkinson's Dis. 2020;10(3):757-74.
6. Radhakrishnan DM, Goyal V. Parkinson's disease: A review. Neurol India. 2018;66:S26-35.
7. EPDA. (2019). Motor symptoms. [online] Available from https://www.epda.eu.com/about-parkinsons/symptoms/motor-symptoms/bradykinesia/. [Last accessed June, 2021].
8. Kim SD, Allen NE, Canning CG, Fung VSC. Postural instability in patients with Parkinson's disease. Epidemiology, pathophysiology and management. CNS Drugs. 2013;27(2):97-112.
9. Editorial Team. (2017). Symptoms—Postural Instability and Balancing Issues. [online] Available from https://parkinsonsdisease.net/symptoms/balancing-issues-postural-instability/. [Last accessed June, 2021].
10. Sung VW, Nicholas AP. Nonmotor symptoms in Parkinson's disease: expanding the view of Parkinson's disease beyond a pure motor, pure dopaminergic problem. Neurol Clin. 2013;31(3 Suppl):S1-16.
11. Hermanowicz N. Impact of non-motor symptoms in Parkinson's disease: a PMD alliance survey. Neuropsychiatr Dis Treat. 2019;15(3):2205-12.
12. Todorova A, Jenner P, Chaudhari KR. Non-motor Parkinson's: integral to motor Parkinson's, yet often neglected. Pract Neurol. 2014;14(2):310-22.
13. Kulisevsky J, Luquin MR, Arbelo JM, Burguera JA, Carrillo F, Castro A, et al. Advanced Parkinson's disease: clinical characteristics and treatment (part 1). Neurología. 2013;28(8):503-21.

CHAPTER 2

Parkinson's Disease: Pathophysiology and Diagnosis

PATHOPHYSIOLOGY

Parkinson's disease (PD) is an elderly disease and is associated with multiple risk factors and genetic mutations. These risk factors often include oxidative stress, free radicals, and various environmental toxins. Some of the risk factors which are associated with PD include:[1]

- Environmental toxins such as:
  - Carbon disulfide
  - Cyanide
  - Herbicides
  - Methanol and organic solvents
  - Pesticides
- Head trauma
- High caloric intake
- Increased body mass index
- Inflammation associated with activation of microglia
- Methcathinone (manganese content)
- Methamphetamine/amphetamine abuse
- Mitochondrial dysfunction
- Nitric oxide toxicity
- *Oxidative stress*:
  - Formation of free radicals (e.g., hydrogen peroxide)
  - Potent neurotoxins (e.g., 1-methyl-4-phenyl-1,2,3,6-tetrahydropyridine)
- Postinfection states

- Signal-mediated apoptosis
- Elevated cholesterol

Gene mutations associated with PD are:[1]
- *Alpha synuclein* (SNCA) gene
- *Eukaryotic translation initiation factor 4 gamma 1* gene (EIF4G1)
- *Glucocerebrosidase (GBA)* gene
- *Leucine-rich repeat kinase 2 (LRRK2)* gene loci
- *PTEN-induced putative kinase 1 (PINK1)* gene loci
- *Superoxide dismutase 2 (SOD2)* gene
- *Vacuolar protein sorting 35 (VPS35) homolog* gene

Parkinson's disease could involve two pathological mechanisms: (1) Premature selective loss of dopamine neurons; and (2) Accumulation of α-synuclein Lewy bodies that are misfolded. Unfortunately, which phase occurs first is not clear. However, what is known is based on many clinical studies that there is progressive degeneration of neurons over the years. **Table 1** depicts the staging of Lewy body deposition.[1]

DIAGNOSIS OF PARKINSON'S DISEASE

UK Prospective Diabetes Study Brain Bank Criteria

Many criteria are available for diagnosing PD, but the most accepted criteria is the one introduced by the UK Prospective Diabetes Study (UKPDS) Brain Bank Criteria.[2]

TABLE 1: Break staging of Lewy body.[1]		
Stage	**Sites affected by Lewy bodies**	**Major symptoms**
I	Dorsal motor nucleus of the vagus nerve and olfactory tract	Constipation and anosmia
II	Locus coeruleus and subcoeruleus complex	Sleep and mood dysfunction
III	Substantia nigra	Motor symptoms of Parkinson's disease
IV–VI	Cortical involvement	Dementia and psychosis

Step 1: Diagnosis of a Parkinsonian syndrome bradykinesia and at least one of the following:
- Muscular rigidity
- Rest tremor (4–6 Hz)
- Postural instability unrelated to primary visual, cerebellar, vestibular, or proprioceptive dysfunction

Step 2: Exclusion criteria for PD:
History of:
- Repeated strokes with stepwise progression
- Repeated head injury
- Antipsychotic or dopamine-depleting drugs
- Definite encephalitis and/or oculogyric crises on no drug treatment
- More than one affected relative
- Sustained remission
- Negative response to large doses of levodopa (if malabsorption excluded)
- Strictly unilateral features after 3 years
- *Other neurological features*: Supranuclear gaze palsy, cerebellar signs, early severe autonomic involvement, Babinski sign, and early severe dementia with disturbances of language, memory, or praxis
- Exposure to known neurotoxin
- Presence of cerebral tumor or communicating hydrocephalus on neuroimaging

Step 3: Supportive criteria for PD:
Three or more required for diagnosis of definite PD:
- Unilateral onset
- Rest tremor present
- Progressive disorder
- Persistent asymmetry affecting the side of onset most
- Excellent response to levodopa
- Severe levodopa-induced chorea

- Levodopa response for over 5 years
- Clinical course of over 10 years

Movement Disorder Society Diagnostic Criteria

The most recent diagnostic criteria for PD patients were released by International Parkinson and Movement Disorder Society (MDS) in 2015. The criteria could be a useful tool in diagnosis of PD patients (**Flowchart 1**).[3]

In the MDS set of criteria, the main criterion for diagnosis of PD is the presence of Parkinsonism, defined as bradykinesia, in combination with either rigidity or resting tremor or both. After confirmation of Parkinsonism and evaluation of "absolute exclusion criteria" (symptoms not present in PD), "red flags" (symptoms atypical for PD), and also "supportive criteria" (symptoms typically or often present in PD), the specialist may diagnose either clinically established PD or clinically probable PD.[4]

The MDS has laid out some exclusion criteria, which include:[4]
- Unequivocal cerebellar abnormalities
- Downward vertical supranuclear gaze palsy or selective slowing of downward vertical saccades
- Within the first 5 years of disease, behavioral variant frontotemporal dementia or primary progressive aphasia is seen
- Parkinsonian features restricted to the lower limbs for >3 years
- Treatment history reveals probability of drug-induced Parkinsonism
- Patients do not respond to high-dose of levodopa
- Unequivocal cortical sensory loss, clear limb ideomotor apraxia, or progressive aphasia
- The neuroimaging reveals normal functioning of presynaptic dopaminergic system

Parkinson's Disease: Pathophysiology and Diagnosis

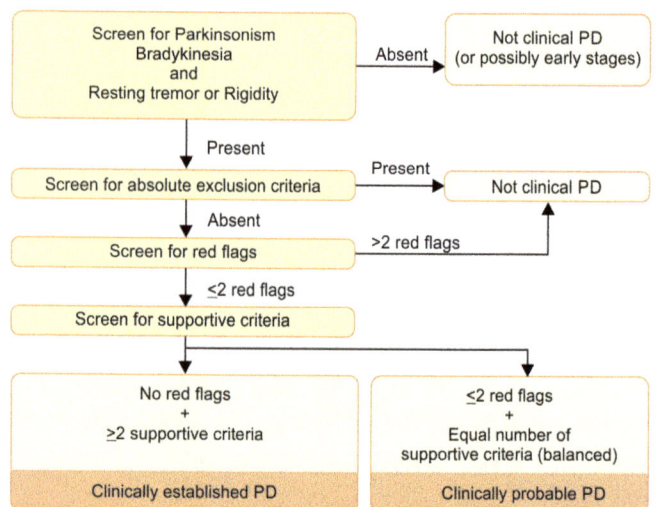

FLOWCHART 1: Summary diagram of Parkinson's disease diagnosis based on the diagnostic criteria of the Movement Disorder Society.[3]

- Alternative conditions which could result in Parkinson's and in connected symptoms

Some of the red flags highlighted in criteria include:[4]
- Within 5 years of onset, the patient is in wheelchair due to progression of gait impairment
- Absence of progression of motor symptoms or signs over >5 years unless stability related to treatment
- *Early bulbar dysfunction*: Severe dysphonia or dysarthria or severe dysphagia within 5 years
- *Inspiratory respiratory dysfunction*: Inspiratory stridor or frequent inspiratory sighs
- *Severe autonomic failure within 5 years of disease onset*:
  - Orthostatic hypotension
  - Severe urinary retention or urinary incontinence not attributable to other condition

- Recurrent (>1 year) falls because of impaired balance within 3 years of onset
- Disproportionate anterocollis (dystonic) or contractures of hand or feet within the first 10 years
- Despite 5 years of disease duration, there is absence of common nonmotor features of diseases is seen, which include sleep dysfunction, autonomic dysfunction, hyposmia, or psychiatric dysfunction
- Otherwise—unexplained pyramidal tract signs, excluding mild reflex asymmetry and isolated extensor plantar response
- Bilateral symmetric Parkinsonism

The supportive criteria include:
- *Clear and dramatic beneficial response to dopaminergic therapy*:
  - Marked improvement with dose increases or marked worsening with dose decreases (>30% in UPDRS III with change in treatment or clearly documented history of marked changes)
  - Marked on/off fluctuations and predictable end-of-dose wearing off
- Levodopa-induced dyskinesia
- Resting tremor of limb
- Either olfactory loss or cardiac sympathetic denervation

MANAGEMENT OF PARKINSON'S DISEASE

The most common strategy for Parkinson's patients is use of medications. The goal with treatment is to rectify the shortage of dopamine, as the deficiency of dopamine is the cause of symptoms. Pharmacological therapy is initiated when symptoms become disabling or disrupt daily activities. Treatments may differ according to the patient's symptoms, age, and responses to specific drugs.[5] It often takes time to find the best combination of drugs for each patient.[6] Management of Parkinson's often varies from drug therapy, surgery, or combination of different treatments (**Table 2**).[7]

Amantadine is often preferred drug in management of PD. Though levodopa is the initial gold standard therapy for PD, its use eventually results in the development of motor fluctuations

TABLE 2: Management of Parkinson's disease (PD)—therapeutic options.[7]

Treatment options	Comments
Dopaminergic medications	• Dopamine agonists available in oral or injection • Often regarded as the gold standard of Parkinson's therapy • Started as first drug in most of patients • L-DOPA and apomorphine
Monoamine oxidase inhibitors (MAOIs), catechol-O-methyl transferase (COMT) inhibitors, and N-methyl-D-aspartate (NMDA) receptor antagonists	• MAOIs such as rasagiline or selegiline • COMT inhibitors such as entacapone • NMDA antagonists such as amantadine and memantine • Inhibit breakdown of levodopa and dopamine through oral drugs • Do not need increased dosage over time • Milder side effects than dopaminergic drugs • May treat L-DOPA-related dyskinesia
Anticholinergics	• Benztropine, biperiden, diphenhydramine, ethopropazine, orphenadrine, procyclidine, and trihexyphenidyl are included in this therapeutic class of drugs • Reduce acetylcholine activity at choline receptors through oral drugs • Rapid absorption, used for tremor-predominant PD • Can be a monotherapy in early stages

and levodopa-induced dyskinesia (LID).[4] Nearly 40% of PD patients develop LID after 4–6 years of levodopa treatment. For patients with PD who have LID, amantadine can maintain its antidyskinetic effect over several years.[8]

SUMMARY

- Parkinson's disease is the disease of elderly people and is associated with multiple risk factors and genetic mutations, though 25% develop PD before 45 years of age.
- Parkinson's disease could involve premature selective loss of dopamine neurons and accumulation of α-synuclein Lewy bodies that are misfolded.
- Bradykinesia is the most important feature.
- Tremor without bradykinesia is not enough for the diagnosis.
- Patients should have a clear effect of their antiparkinsonian medications, if the dose is sufficient.
- Treatment goal is to rectify the shortage of dopamine, as the deficiency of dopamine is the cause of symptoms.
- Amantadine is often preferred over levodopa.

REFERENCES

1. Pradahan M, Srivastava R. Etiology. Epidemiology, Diagnosis and Current Therapeutic Protocols for Parkinson's Disease (PD): An Overview. Med Surg Radiol. 2020;5(1):A186-91.
2. National Collaborating Centre for Chronic Conditions (UK). Parkinson's Disease: National Clinical Guideline for Diagnosis and Management in Primary and Secondary Care. London: Royal College of Physicians; 2006.
3. Postuma RB, Berg D, Stern M, Poewe W, Olanow CW, Oertel W, et al. MDS clinical diagnostic criteria for Parkinson's disease. Mov Disord. 2015;30(12):1591-601.
4. Pirtošek Z, Bajenaru O, Kovács N, Milanov I, Relja M, Skorvanek M. Update on the Management of Parkinson's Disease for General Neurologists. Parkinsons Dis. 2020;2020:9131474.

5. Goldenberg MM. Medical management of Parkinson's disease. PT. 2008;33(10):590-606.
6. American Association of Neurological Surgeons. (2021). Parkinson's disease. [online] Available from https://www.aans.org/en/Patients/Neurosurgical-Conditions-and-Treatments/Parkinsons-Disease. [Last accessed June, 2021].
7. Lee TK, Yankee EK. A review on Parkinson's disease treatment. Neuroimmunol Neuroinflamm. 2021;8:10.
8. Brooks M. (2014). Amantadine Has Lasting Benefit on Levodopa-Induced Dyskinesia. [online] Available from https://www.medscape.com/viewarticle/818839. [Last accessed June, 2021].

CHAPTER 3

Role of Amantadine in Parkinson's Disease

INTRODUCTION AND BASIC CHEMISTRY

In 1966, amantadine was first approved as an antiviral compound by the Food and Drug Administration (FDA). Later in 1968, a 58-year-old woman with moderately severe Parkinson's disease had remarkable remission in her symptoms of rigidity, tremor, and akinesia when initiated on amantadine.

The drug is hydrophilic in nature and penetrates the blood–brain barrier (due to active transport probably via a proton-coupled organic cation antiporter). Amantadine is a symmetrical C10 primary amine with a remarkable cyclic structure belonging to the class of aminoadamantanes (see **Fig. 1**).[1,2]

- Amantadine is a synthetic tricyclic amine that belongs to the class of aminoadamantanes
- It is an antiparkinsonian agent and anti-influenzal virostatic drug

PHARMACODYNAMIC

Amantadine is an oral N-methyl-D-aspartate (NMDA) receptor antagonist, which was originally approved as an antiviral and was later

- Amantadine is an oral NMDA receptor antagonist
- Amantadine improves bradykinesia, rigidity, and tremor
- Amantadine has antidyskinetic effects

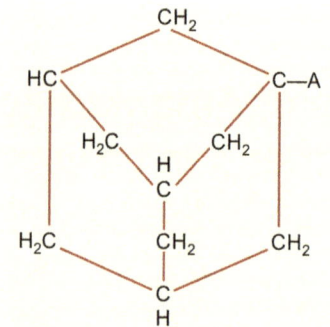

FIG. 1: Structure of amantadine.

discovered to exert an antiparkinsonian effect with remissions in rigidity, bradykinesia, and tremor.[3]

MECHANISM OF ACTION OF AMANTADINE

Amantadine, a tricyclic amine, exhibits both dopaminergic and nondopaminergic actions, owing to its well absorption and is largely excreted unchanged in the urine.[3,4] Amantadine has several proposed mechanisms of action (see **Fig. 2**).[4]

General Pharmacodynamics of Amantadine:[5]

- *Dopaminergic system*: Amantadine inhibiting dopamine reuptake in synaptic cleft and increases dopamine level in the brain. These effects are observed at clinically high doses in humans. Though exact effect on dopaminergic transmission are still unknown, some results show that amantadine exhibits direct effects on D2 receptors. However, in one of the studies among patients, being treated with amantadine 200 mg/day and were suspended L-DOPA treatment a night before, showed an increase in ^{11}C raclopride binding in the caudate and putamen. Thereby, suggesting that amantadine increased neosynthesis of D2 receptors.[5]

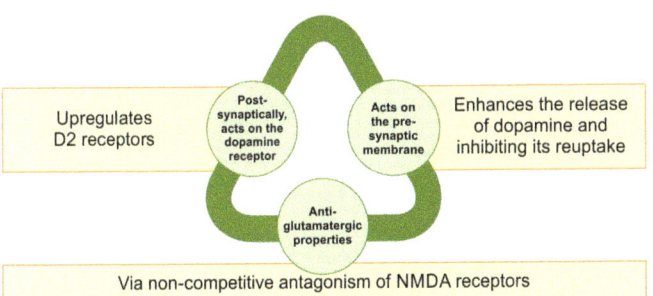

FIG. 2: Amantadine mechanism of action. (NMDA: N-methyl-D-aspartate)

- *Noradrenergic system*: The drug exerts similar pharmacodynamic actions to that of tricyclic antidepressants, thereby causing a significant increase in the levels of norepinephrine.[5]
- *Glutamatergic system*: Amantadine also has noncompetitive NMDA receptor antagonist. It inhibits NMDA receptor activation through the stabilization of ion channels and more rapid channel closure.[5] The mechanism of action is owing to its NMDA blockade action (see **Fig. 3**).[6]

- Amantadine is indicated in the treatment of Parkinson's disease both as a monotherapy as well as in combination with levodopa
- In addition, the drug is used for other indications which include drug-induced extrapyramidal side effects, attention deficit disorder, L-DOPA-induced motor fluctuations, traumatic brain injury, and autistic spectrum disorders

- *Immunomodulation:* Additionally, the drug also has immunomodulatory effects. In patients with Parkinson's disease, the interleukin (IL)-2 is dysfunctional and amantadine restores the production of IL-2. Various clinical studies have shown that treatment with amantadine was an independent predictor of improved survival in Parkinson's disease.[5]

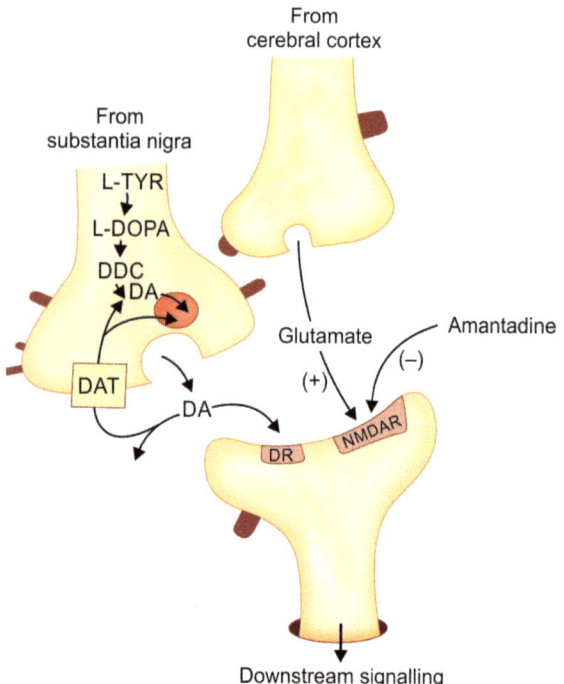

FIG. 3: Interface between a dopaminergic (DAergic) nigrostriatal nerve terminal in which dopamine (DA) is synthesized from L-tyrosine (L-Tyr) via L-DOPA to DA with a glutamatergic terminal of the corticostriatal tract and the postsynaptic neuron.[6]

Of all these proposed mechanisms of action, NMDA receptor blocking activity could be more relevant mechanism therapeutically for relevant doses of amantadine.[5]

CLINICAL INDICATIONS

Amantadine is indicated in the treatment of Parkinsonism and drug-induced extrapyramidal reactions, which include but not limited to:[7]

- Idiopathic Parkinson's disease
- Postencephalitic Parkinsonism
- Symptomatic Parkinsonism followed by carbon monoxide intoxication, drugs, etc.
- Vascular Parkinsonism in association with cerebral arteriosclerosis
- Drug-induced Parkinsonism

PHARMACOKINETIC PROPERTIES

After oral administration, amantadine is well absorbed, and maximum plasma level is attained at approximately 3.3 hours after administration. The drug has a half-life of approximately 16 hours. Additionally, almost 90% of the drug is excreted unchanged in urine. The approved clinical dose is 100 mg twice daily, which based on the need can be increased up to 400 mg/day.[5]

In a clinical study, 24 healthy adult male volunteers were evaluated for amantadine pharmacokinetic profile. The volunteers were administered oral single dose of amantadine hydrochloride. Following findings were reported in the study:[7]

Maximum plasma concentration was 0.22 ± 0.03 µg/mL
Time to peak concentration was 3.3 ± 1.5 hours
Oral clearance was 0.28 ± 0.11 L/h/kg
Half-life was 17 ± 4 hours

However, in another study on six healthy volunteers and six elderly volunteers, single oral dose of amantadine 200 mg reported amantadine presence in nasal mucous after 4 and 6 hours of dosing with 67% bound to plasma proteins.[7]

Clearance of amantadine is significantly reduced in adults with renal insufficiency and elimination half-life increases >two- to threefold when creatinine clearance is <40 mL/min. Amantadine half-life may be 8 days in patients on chronic maintenance hemodialysis. Amantadine is nondialysable and maintains blood level even after dialysis.[7]

A detailed breakdown of amantadine pharmacokinetics has been depicted in **Table 1**.[3,8]

TABLE 1: Pharmacokinetic properties of amantadine.		
Absorption	Bioavailability	Good GI absorption; Peak plasma in 2–4 h
	Onset	Within 48 h
	Plasma concentrations	• Peak plasma concentrations attained at 200 mg daily of <1,000 ng/mL • Dosage > 200 mg results in greater than proportional increase in peak plasma
	Special populations	Increased in renal impairment
Distribution		Distributed into nasal secretions, erythrocytes, CSF, and milk
	Plasma protein binding	67%
Elimination	Metabolism	Undergoes N-acetylation
	Elimination route	• Excreted unchanged in urine • 5–15% excreted in urine as acetylamantadine
	Half-life	16 h
	Renal impairment patients	18.5–81.3 h
	Chronic hemodialysis	8.3 days
	Geriatric adults	29 h

(CSF: cerebrospinal fluid; GI: gastrointestinal)

Metabolism

Pharmacokinetic studies have revealed eight amantadine metabolites. One of the metabolites, an N-acetylated compound was accounted for 5–15% of the administered dose. In 5 of 12 healthy volunteers, plasma acetylamantadine accounted for up to 80% of the concurrent amantadine plasma concentration following ingestion of 200 mg dose of amantadine. However, in remaining seven volunteers, no acetylamantadine was detected in plasma. The contribution of this metabolite to efficacy or toxicity is not known.[9]

There exists a relationship between plasma amantadine concentration and its toxicity. As concentration increases, toxicity seems to be more prevalent; however, absolute values of amantadine concentrations associated with adverse effects have not been fully defined.[9]

Elimination

Amantadine is primarily excreted unchanged in the urine by glomerular filtration and tubular secretion (**Table 2**).

A study on 19 health volunteers reported plasma half-life of 16 ± 6 hours (range: 9–31 h). In another study with 15 healthy volunteers, plasma amantadine clearance ranged from 0.2 to 0.3 L/h/kg after the administration of 5–25 mg intravenous doses. In six healthy volunteers, the ratio of amantadine renal clearance to apparent oral plasma clearance was 0.79 ± 0.17 (mean ± SD).[9]

TABLE 2: Amantadine clearance and half-life.	
Parameters	Value
Oral clearance	0.28 ± 0.11 L/h/kg (range: 0.14–0.62 L/h/kg)
Half-life	17 ± 4 h (range: 10–25 h)

The apparent oral plasma clearance of amantadine is reduced, and the plasma half-life and plasma concentrations are increased in healthy elderly individuals aged 60 years and older. In another study with seven healthy, elderly male volunteers, the apparent plasma clearance of amantadine was 0.10 ± 0.04 L/h/kg (range: 0.06–0.17 L/h/kg) and the half-life was 29 ± 7 hours (range: 20–41 h) with single amantadine dose administration of 25–75 mg. However, the reason for changes could be due to decline in renal function or could be age related which is not known. In a study of young healthy subjects ($n = 20$), mean renal clearance of amantadine, normalized for body mass index, was 1.5-fold higher in males compared to females ($p < 0.032$). Compared with otherwise healthy adult individuals, the clearance of amantadine is significantly reduced in adult patients with renal impairment. In patients on chronic maintenance hemodialysis, with creatinine clearance < 40 mL/min/1.73 m^2, there is an increase in the elimination half-life by two- to threefold. During hemodialysis, amantadine is removed in negligible amounts. Urine pH has an influence on excretion of amantadine; therefore, the excretion rate of amantadine increases when urine is acidic. Administration of urine-acidifying drugs may increase the elimination of the drug from the body.[9]

SUMMARY

- Amantadine is a synthetic tricyclic amine that belongs to the class of aminoadamantanes having an NMDA receptor antagonist activity.
- It is an antiparkinsonian agent and virostatic anti-influenza drug.
- Amantadine improves bradykinesia, rigidity, and tremor and has antidyskinetic effects.
- Amantadine increases norepinephrine levels and has pharmacological actions that are like those of tricyclic antidepressants.

- Amantadine may also have immunomodulatory properties. It restored the production of interleukin (IL)-2, which is dysfunctional in patients with Parkinson's disease.
- Amantadine is well absorbed orally and attains maximum concentration at approximately 3.3 hours.
- Amantadine has half-life of approximately 16 hours and approximately 90% of amantadine is excreted unchanged in urine.
- The usual clinical dose of amantadine is 100 mg twice daily, which can be increased up to 400 mg/day.

REFERENCES

1. Hesselink KMJ. Amantadine and phenytoin: patent protected cases of drug repositioning. Clin Investig. 2017;7(1):11-6.
2. Perez-Lloret S, Rascol O. Efficacy and safety of amantadine for the treatment of L-DOPA-induced dyskinesia. J Neural Transm (Vienna). 2018;125(8):1237-50.
3. Sharma VD, Lyons KE, Pahwa R. Amantadine extended-release capsules for levodopa-induced dyskinesia in patients with Parkinson's disease. Ther Clin Risk Manag. 2018;14(3):665-73.
4. Warren N. The Use of Amantadine in Parkinson's Disease and other Akinetic-Rigid Disorders. ACNR. 2004;4(5):37-41.
5. Raupp-Barcaro IF, Vital MA, Galduróz JC, Andreatini R. Potential antidepressant effect of amantadine: a review of preclinical studies and clinical trials. Braz J Psychiatry. 2018;40(4):449-58.
6. Butterworth RF. Amantadine Treatment for Parkinson's Disease during COVID-19: Bimodal Action Targeting Viral Replication and the NMDA Receptor. J Parkinsons Dis Alzheimer Dis. 2020;7(1):4.
7. Drugs.com. (2019). Amantadine. [online] Available from https://www.drugs.com/pro/amantadine.html#s-34090-1. [Last accessed June, 2021].
8. Drugs.com. (2019). Amantadine. [online] Available from https://www.drugs.com/monograph/amantadine.html#pharmacokinetics. [Last accessed June, 2021].
9. Ciplamed. (2019). Amantrel capsules. [online] Available from https://www.ciplamed.com/content/amantrel-capsules. [Last accessed June, 2021].

CHAPTER 4

Clinical Efficacy and Safety of Amantadine

EFFICACY OF AMANTADINE IN LEVODOPA-INDUCED DYSKINESIA IN PARKINSON'S DISEASE

Amantadine and the Risk of Dyskinesia in Patients with Early Parkinson's Disease

Levodopa has been the most prescribed drugs in Parkinson's disease (PD). However, the drug has been associated with motor and psychiatric side effects,[1] one of which is levodopa-induced dyskinesia (LID). Nearly 50% of PD patients develop LID within 5 years of treatment with levodopa,[2] owing to which a lot of interest has been gone to alternative drugs with improved side effect profiles and potential to replace or augment levodopa therapy.[1] It has been noted that onset of LID could be delayed among patients with use of dopamine agonist; however, the option comes with other adverse effects.[2] Amantadine, which was initially prescribed as an antiviral drug, has now been widely used in PD, owing to its improvement in symptoms and better safety profile.[1] In addition, amantadine has significant clinical data supporting its antidyskinetic effects.[2]

- Nearly 50% of PD patients develop LID within 5 years of treatment with levodopa.[2]
- Amantadine as an initial treatment could decrease the incidence of dyskinesia in drug-naïve PD patients.[2]

TABLE 1: Study design.[2]

Group A-1	Phase 1 amantadine	Phase 2 levodopa	
Group A-2	Phase 1 amantadine	Phase 1.5 dopamine agonist	Phase 2 levodopa
Group B	Phase 1 dopamine agonists	Phase 2 levodopa	

In the study, patients were divided into three treatment groups: Group A-1, Group A-2, and Group B (**Table 1**). Group A-1 patients were started on amantadine 150–300 mg thrice daily and levodopa was added on the need basis. Group A-2 patients were started on amantadine, dopamine agonist, when needed, and levodopa, whereas patients in Group B were started on dopamine agonists followed by levodopa as and when required. Amantadine was only prescribed to these patients when patients developed dyskinesia.[2]

Results from the study reported that patients in Group A-1 and Group A-2 tended to develop dyskinesia less when compared with those in Group B. Overall, only 8.93% of patients developed dyskinesia for 30 months follow-up period. Amantadine as an initial treatment could decrease the incidence of dyskinesia in drug-naïve PD patients. Therefore, it could be concluded that amantadine at initial stages of PD could avoid a direct effect on postsynaptic dopaminergic receptors so that pulsatile stimulation could be reduced when compared to using levodopa as an initial treatment.[2]

Efficacy and Safety of Amantadine for the Treatment of Levodopa-induced Dyskinesia

Amantadine is available in various dosage forms and various clinical trials have been conducted to evaluate its efficacy and safety in PD patients.[3]

- Study conducted by Verhagen Metman in 1998 reported 35% improvement in Unified Parkinson's Disease Rating Scale (UPDRS) Part IV and Abnormal Involuntary Movement Scale (AIMS) with amantadine 300–400 mg for 3 weeks. Amantadine substantially ameliorates LID peak-dose dyskinesias without a concomitant worsening of Parkinsonian symptoms, which were related to plasma amantadine concentration.[4]
- 56% lower AIMS score was reported with amantadine at an average dose of 362 mg for 7–10 days.[3]
- Amantadine 200 mg for 3 weeks exhibited 45% reduction in UPDRS IV scores and 64% reduction in Rush Dyskinesia Rating Scale (RDRS).[3]
- Study conducted by Pahwa et al. reported extended-release amantadine at a dose of 274 mg for 25 weeks exhibited >twofold reduction in Unified Dyskinesia Rating Scale (UDysRS) and additionally reduced off-time.[3]
- Similarly, 42% reduction in Movement Disorder Society (MDS)-UPDRS IV score was reported in a dose of amantadine 274 mg up to 88 weeks.[3]
- These clinical studies reported constipation, cardiovascular dysfunction including QT prolongation, orthostatic hypotension and edema, neuropsychiatric symptoms such as hallucinations, confusion and delirium, nausea, and livedo reticularis as the most common adverse reactions with amantadine.[3]
- In an acute double-blind placebo-controlled study, L-DOPA followed by amantadine treatment improved dyskinesias by 50% with no loss of benefit for the motor symptoms in patients with peak-dose dyskinesias. When compared with placebo, amantadine overtime significantly reduced dyskinesia.[5]

- Amantadine substantially ameliorates LID peak-dose dyskinesias without a concomitant worsening of Parkinsonian symptoms.[4]

POSTURAL REFLEX IMPAIRMENT IN PARKINSON'S DISEASE

Postural instability is one of the cardinal features of PD together with rest tremor, rigidity, and bradykinesia.[6] Since PD affects the reflexes required for standing, which gets unstable in postural instability. This results in person falling backward when slightly jostled, thereby resulting in increased chances of falling.[7] Within 2 years of PD diagnosis, nearly 34% of patients develop postural instability, which increases to 71% in 10 years and 92% at 15 years.[6]

Study conducted by Chan et al. in a prospective multicenter observational study evaluated the efficacy of amantadine in PD patients with axial symptoms such as speech, gait, and balance impairment. Treatment with amantadine significantly improved postural stability (item 30) in patients with advanced PD. From the study, it was concluded that amantadine treatment resulted in subjective improvement in speech, gait, or balance among 76.1% of patients whereas 65.2% of patients reported improvement in gait and balance. Thereby, suggesting amantadine could be beneficial on axial symptoms in PD patients.[8]

- Amantadine treatment significantly improved postural stability (item 30) in patients with advanced PD.[8]
- Amantadine may have new beneficial effects on axial symptoms in PD patients with STN-DBS.[8]
- Amantadine is associated with self-reported improvement in FOG in patients with PD.[10]

EFFICACY OF AMANTADINE IN FREEZING OF GAIT

Freezing of gait (FOG) is one of the typical gait disorders observed in PD. The condition is defined as an onset of inability to start effective steps without known cause and is most experienced during step initiation and turning, especially facing with obstacles, doorways, stress, and distraction. It is estimated to affect nearly 7% of the people with early disease and more than half of patients with advanced PD leading to loss of quality, independence, and mobility. Amantadine could exert clinical benefits independent to dopaminergic mechanism.[9] Amantadine 100 mg twice daily for duration of 20 months improved FOG symptoms in 10 out of 11 patients (**Table 2**).[10]

Amantadine dose (mg)	Duration of treatment (months)	Response	Reduced response	Adverse events
100 daily	66	+		
100 BID	15	–		
100 BID	20	+		
100 BID	36	+		
100 BID	23	+	√	
100 BID	19	+	√	
100 BID	40	+		Blurred vision
100 BID	6	+	√	Lower extremity edema
100 BID	7	+	√	
100 BID	46	+		
100 BID	7	+		Hallucinations

TABLE 2: Summary of freezing of gait response to amantadine.[10]

[BID: twice daily; (+): improvement in freezing of gait; (–): worsening of freezing of gait]

Clinical Efficacy and Safety of Amantadine

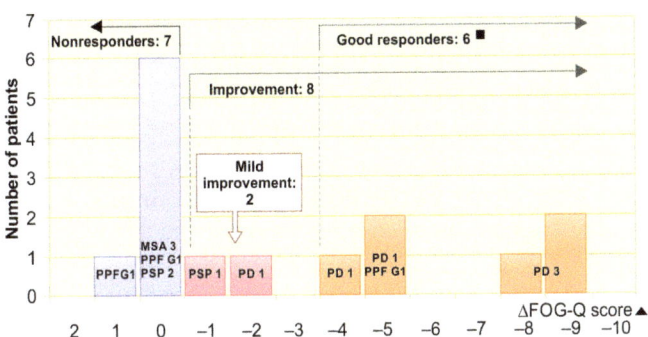

(FOG-Q: Freezing of Gait Questionnaire; MSA: multiple system atrophy; PD: Parkinson's disease; PPFG: primary progressive freezing gait; PSP: progressive supranuclear palsy)

FIG. 1: Improvement in FOG-Q score.

In another study, improvement in Freezing of Gait Questionnaire (FOG-Q) score was seen in eight patients (53.3%) and a marked improvement was seen in six patients [five with PD and one with primary progressive freezing gait (PPFG)] (**Fig. 1**).[11]

- Amantadine may be effective in FOG resistant to dopaminergic drugs. The improvement was seen mainly in PD.[11]

DURATION OF AMANTADINE BENEFIT ON DYSKINESIA OF SEVERE PARKINSON'S DISEASE

A double-blind study for the duration of 12 months evaluated the duration of benefits on dyskinesia in PD patients. The study reported that after 15 days therapy with amantadine, there was reduction by 45% in the total dyskinesia scores.[12,13]

AMANTADINE EFFECTIVENESS IN MULTIPLE SYSTEM ATROPHY AND PROGRESSIVE SUPRANUCLEAR PALSY

Progressive supranuclear palsy (PSP) is a neurodegenerative disease characterized by Parkinsonism with prominent axial involvement and postural reflex abnormality, bulbar symptoms, supranuclear ophthalmoplegia, and higher cortical dysfunction.[14,15]

Amantadine treatment was given to 14 PSP patients (three females, 11 males) in which six patients (42.9%) had some improvement whereas five patients (35.7%) had no benefit (**Table 3**).[16]

Amantadine treatment was given to 13 multiple system atrophy (MSA) patients (six females, seven males) in which eight patients (61.5%) improved whereas four patients (30.8%) did not benefit (**Table 4**).[16]

- 300 mg amantadine reduces dyskinesia in Parkinson's disease by approximately 45%, but the benefit lasted <8 months.[12]

Improvement is likely related to N-methyl-D-aspartate (NMDA) antagonist properties of amantadine. The authors recommend consideration of amantadine in the management of both PSP and MSA.[16]

How long to use amantadine: Long-term data?

Zeldowicz et al. conducted a dual study to evaluate the long-term benefits of amantadine without concomitant levodopa and the advantages of combined amantadine and levodopa over single-drug therapy. In the study, 19 patients were given amantadine for a mean duration of 21 months—11 for over 2 years, 5 for 8–20 months, and 3 for 6 months.[17]

The study at the end of long-term amantadine reported improvement in functional and neurological deficits:[17]

TABLE 3: Improvement with amantadine therapy in PSP patients.

PS stage* at Amd initiation	Response to Amd	Deceased (D) or currently followed (F)
3.5	Imp hand function	D
2	No imp	F
2	No imp	F
3	No Imp	D (autopsy)
3	Imp	F
2	Imp	F
3	Imp	F
Unknown	Unknown	D (autopsy)
2	No progression for 1.5 years	D (autopsy)
2	Unknown	Unknown
3	Imp deteriorate after withdrawal 7 years later	D
3	No imp	Unknown
2	No imp–"made symptoms worse"	D (autopsy)
1	Unknown	D (autopsy)

*Hoehn and Yahr stage.

(Amd: amantadine; BR: bradykinesia; F: female; Imp: improvement; M: male; N/A: not applicable; PS: Parkinsonism; PSP: progressive supranuclear palsy)

- Mean reduction in functional deficit in the four activities ranged from 57.3 to 64.7% (**Table 5**)
- Mean reduction in neurological deficit in the five signs ranged from 67.0 to 92.7%
- Significant improvement in symptoms was also reported in the study (**Table 6**)

TABLE 4: Improvement with amantadine therapy in MSA patients.

PS stage* at Amd initiation	Response to Amd	Amd side effects	Deceased (D) or currently followed (f)
4.5	Imp RIG - no longer bed-ridden; can feed self	"Dizziness" but also taking LD	D (autopsy)
5	Imp RIG, BR upper limbs	None	D
3	"Paralyzed legs" upon withdrawal	Leg edema	Moved out of province
4	No imp	Hallucinations	D
3	Imp BR, RIG, ambulation	None	F
3	No imp	None	D
3	Unknown	Unknown	D
2	Imp–DK	None	D (autopsy)
4	Imp–RT, RIG, BR; ADL's	None	D (autopsy)
3	No progression for at least 1 year	None	D (autopsy)
3	Imp BR, RIG	None	D (autopsy)
5	No imp	None	D (autopsy)
5	No imp	None	D

*Hoehn and Yahr stage.

(Amd: amantadine; BR: bradykinesia; F: female; Imp: improvement; M: male; MSA: multiple system atrophy; N/A: not applicable; PS: Parkinsonism; RIG: rigidity; RT: resting tremor)

Over a mean duration of 21 months, all 19 patients continued improvement without any signs of decline in effects of amantadine.[17]

TABLE 5: Improvement in functional level.

	Walking	Dressing	Feeding	Toiletry
Mean improvement (%)	61.1	58.7	57.3	64.7

Point scores: 0 = no symptoms, 4 = maximum disability.
Note: None of patients scored worse on any of the four indicators when on medication.

TABLE 6: Improvement in symptoms.

	Tremor	Rigidity	Akinesia	Speech	Salivation
Mean improvement (%)	69	67.1	68.6	67.0	92.7

Point scores: 0 = no symptoms, 4 = maximum disability.
Note: Not a single patient obtained a worse score on medication on any of the five indicators.

USE OF AMANTADINE IN OTHER DISORDERS

Amantadine as an Antiviral Agent

Amantadine was first approved to be used as an antiviral compound, which specifically inhibits replication of influenza A virus at a micromolar concentration.[18] The drug inhibits replication of influenza A virus by interfering with the uncoating of the virus inside the cell. Amantadine is an M2 inhibitor, which blocks the ion channel formed by the M2 protein that spans the viral membrane.[19]

Owing to lack of potential benefits of amantadine, the drug has not been used widely. Therefore, review was conducted to assess the efficacy and safety of amantadine in healthy adults. The study reported that amantadine prevented: 25% of influenza-like illness (ILI) cases [95% confidence interval (CI) 13–36%] and 61% of influenza A cases (95% CI 35–76%). The review concluded that amantadine has comparable efficacy and effectiveness in relieving or treating symptoms of influenza A in healthy adults.[20]

Amantadine in the Management of Ataxia

Degenerative cerebellar ataxias (CAs) are a group of disorders associated with progressive degeneration of the cerebellum, and its afferent and efferent pathways, resulting in the impairment of both appendicular and axial motor control. Patients often present with complaints of clumsiness, speech changes, and unsteady gait.[21]

Youn et al. conducted a short-term, open-label preliminary study to evaluate the benefits of amantadine in patients with probable MSA with predominant CA. The study recruited 20 patients.[22]

The study concluded that treatment with amantadine:[22]
- Significantly decreased severity of ataxia from 42.5 to 37.3 ($p < 0.001$)
- Duration of the effect lasted >1 month
- No side effects were reported

Though mechanism of amantadine is not clear from the study, it was concluded that amantadine treatment can be a safe management option in CA.[22]

Amantadine in the Management of Traumatic Brain Injury

Traumatic brain injury (TBI) is defined as a disruption in the normal function of the brain that can be caused by a bump, blow, or jolt to the head or penetrating head injury.[23] Severe TBI is associated with decreased attention, memory problems, confusion and impulsiveness, weakness, and impaired coordination and balance.[24] The treatment goals for TBI are to improve arousal through modulation of the dopaminergic or noradrenergic pathways damaged during the injury. Amantadine exhibits both dopaminergic agonist and NMDA antagonist activity because of which could be beneficial in patients with severe TBI.[25]

In a double-blind, randomized controlled clinical trial, patients were randomized to receive amantadine and placebo for the duration of 4 weeks. The study reported:[25]

- The rate of recovery, as measured by the Disability Rating Scale, was found to be greater in the treatment arm as compared with the placebo arm (difference in slope –0.24 point/week, $p = 0.007$) over the 4-week treatment interval.
- A greater percentage of patients reached key behavioral milestones in the amantadine group compared with placebo.

SUMMARY

- Amantadine could decrease the incidence of dyskinesia in drug-naïve PD patients.
- Amantadine treatment improved dyskinesias by 50% with no loss of benefit for the motor symptoms in patients.
- Amantadine is associated with self-reported improvement in FOG in PD patients.
- Amantadine could be beneficial on axial symptoms in PD patients.
- Amantadine may be effective in FOG resistant to dopaminergic drugs.
- Amantadine could be beneficial in MSA and PSP patients owing to its NMDA antagonist properties.
- Long-term amantadine reported improvement in functional and neurological deficits.
- In addition to its benefits in PD, amantadine has shown clinical benefits in influenza A virus, ataxia, and has a potential role in management of TBI.

REFERENCES

1. Crosby N, Deane KH, Clarke CE. Amantadine in Parkinson's disease. Cochrane Database Syst Rev. 2003;(1):CD003468.
2. Kim A, Kim YE, Yun JY, Kim HJ, Yang HJ, Lee WW, et al. Amantadine and the Risk of Dyskinesia in Patients with Early Parkinson's Disease: An Open-Label, Pragmatic Trial. J Mov Disord. 2018;11(2):65-71.
3. Perez-Lloret S, Rascol O. Efficacy and safety of amantadine for the treatment of L-DOPA-induced dyskinesia. J Neural Transm (Vienna). 2018;125(8):1237-50.
4. Metman LV, Dotto PD, van den Munckhof P, Fang J, Mouradian MM, Chase TN. Amantadine as treatment for dyskinesias and motor fluctuations in Parkinson's disease. Neurology. 1998;50(5):1323-6.
5. Dotto PD, Pavese N, Gambaccini G, Bernardini S, Metman LV, Chase TN, et al. Intravenous amantadine improves levadopa-induced dyskinesias: an acute double-blind placebo-controlled study. Mov Disord. 2001;16(3):515-20.
6. Kim SD, Allen NE, Canning CG, Fung VSC. Postural instability in patients with Parkinson's disease. Epidemiology, pathophysiology and management. CNS Drugs. 2013;27(2):97-112.
7. Editorial Team. (2017). Symptoms—Postural Instability and Balancing Issues. [online] Available from https://parkinsonsdisease.net/symptoms/balancing-issues-postural-instability/. [Last accessed June, 2021].
8. Chan HF, Kukkle PL, Merello M, Lim SY, Poon YY, Moro E. Amantadine improves gait in PD patients with STN stimulation. Parkinsonism Relat Disord. 2013;19(3):316-9.
9. Zhang LL, Canning SD, Wang XP. Freezing of Gait in Parkinsonism and its Potential Drug Treatment. Curr Neuropharmacol. 2016;14(4):302-6.
10. Malkani R, Zadikoff C, Melen O, Videnovic A, Borushko E, Simuni T. Amantadine for freezing of gait in patients with Parkinson's disease. Clin Neuropharmacol. 2012;35(6):266-8.
11. Kim YE, Yun JY, Jeon BS. Effect of intravenous amantadine on dopaminergic-drug-resistant freezing of gait. Parkinsonism Relat Disord. 2011;17(6):491-2.
12. Thomas A, Lacono D, Luciano A, Armellino K, Di I, Onofrj M. Duration of amantadine benefit on dyskinesia of severe Parkinson's disease. J Neurol Neurosurg Psychiatry. 2004;75(1):141-3.
13. Kompoliti K, Goetz CG, Litvan I, Jellinger K, Verny M. Pharmacological therapy in progressive supranuclear palsy. Arch Neurol. 1998;55(8):1099-102.

14. The MSA Coalition. (2020). Multiple System Atrophy (MSA). [online] Available from https://www.multiplesystematrophy.org/about-msa/. [Last accessed June, 2021].
15. National Organization for Rare Disorders (NORD). (2021). Multiple System Atrophy. [online] Available from https://rarediseases.org/rare-diseases/multiple-system-atrophy/. [Last accessed June, 2021].
16. Rajrut AH, Uitti RJ, Fenton ME, George D. Amantadine effectiveness in multiple system atrophy and progressive supranuclear palsy. Parkinsonism Relat Disord. 1997;3(4):211-4.
17. Zeldowicz LR, Huberman J. Long-term therapy of Parkinson's disease with amantadine, alone and combined with levodopa. Can Med Assoc J. 1973;109(7):588-93.
18. Butterworth RF. Amantadine Treatment for Parkinson's Disease during COVID-19: Bimodal Action Targeting Viral Replication and the NMDA Receptor. J Parkinsons Dis Alzheimer Dis. 2020;7(1):7.
19. Kamps BS, Hoffmann C. (2009). Amantadine. [online] Available from http://www.influenzareport.com/ir/drugs/amanta.htm. [Last accessed June, 2021].
20. Jefferson T, Demicheli V, Pietrantonj CD, Rivetti D. Amantadine and rimantadine for influenza A in adults. Cochrane Database Syst Rev. 2006;2006(2):CD001169.
21. Sarva H, Shanker VL. (2014). Treatment Options in Degenerative Cerebellar Ataxia: A Systematic Review. [online] Available from https://www.movementdisorders.org/MDS/Journals/Clinical-Practice-E-Journal-Overview/Movement-Disorders-Clinical-Practice-E-Journal-Volume-1-Issue-4/Treatment-Options-in-Degenerative-Cerebellar-Ataxia-A-Systematic-Review.htm. [Last accessed June, 2021].
22. Youn J, Shin H, Kim JS, Cho JW. Preliminary study of intravenous amantadine treatment for ataxia management in patients with probable multiple system atrophy with predominant cerebellar ataxia. J Mov Disord. 2012;5(1):1-4.
23. Centers for Disease Control and Prevention (CDC). (2021). Symptoms of Mild TBI and Concussion. [online] Available from https://www.cdc.gov/traumaticbraininjury/symptoms.html. [Last accessed June, 2021].
24. Traumatic brain injury. Available from: https://www.mayoclinic.org/diseases-conditions/traumatic-brain-injury/symptoms-causes/syc-20378557 [Last accessed June, 2021].
25. Spritzer SD, Kinney CL, Condie J, Wellik KE, Snyder CRH, Wingerchuk DM, et al. Amantadine for patients with severe traumatic brain injury: a critically appraised topic. Neurologist. 2015;19(2):61-4.

CHAPTER 5

Amantadine: Dosage, Adverse Effects, and Drug–Drug Interactions

DOSAGE AND ADMINISTRATION

Dosage for Parkinson's Disease

Adults

Amantadine, when used alone, is prescribed at a dose of 100 mg twice daily and within 48 hours its onset of action takes place. In patients with congestive heart failure, peripheral edema, orthostatic hypotension, or impaired renal function, dosage of amantadine needs reduction.[1]

The initial dose of amantadine is 100 mg daily for patients with associated medical illness or who are already receiving other antiparkinsonian drugs. In patients, who do not respond to amantadine, 100 mg can be increased to 200 mg with a maximum dose of 400 mg daily in a divided dose. However, it is important that patients be under physician supervision in such cases.[1]

Patients who experience benefit from amantadine initially can have decreased effectiveness after a few months. Benefit may be regained by increasing the dose to 300 mg daily. A decision to use other antiparkinsonian drugs may be required.[1]

Dosage for Concomitant Therapy

Additional benefit may be produced when given in concomitant with other antiparkinsonian drugs. Rapid therapeutic benefits are noticed when amantadine and levodopa are initiated concurrently in some patients. In such cases, dose of amantadine should be constantly held at 100 mg daily or twice daily while levodopa dose could be increased gradually for optimal benefits. Addition of amantadine to well tolerated dose of levodopa can result in decrease of treatment fluctuations, which is seen occasionally in patients on levodopa alone. Patients who require a reduction in their usual dose of levodopa because of the development of side effects may possibly regain lost benefits with the addition of amantadine.[1]

Dosage for Drug-induced Extrapyramidal Reactions

As mentioned earlier, the usual dose of amantadine is 100 mg twice daily. Occasionally, some patients may benefit from an increase up to 300 mg daily in divided doses when 200 mg amantadine is not optimal (**Table 1**).[1]

OVERDOSAGE OF AMANTADINE

- The lowest reported acute lethal dose: 1 g.[2]
- Overdosage results in cardiac, respiratory, renal, or central nervous system toxicity.[3]
- *Signs and symptoms*: Neuromuscular disturbances and symptoms of acute psychosis are prominent features of acute poisoning with amantadine.[3]

TABLE 1: Amantadine dosage	
Indications	Dosage
Adult dosage in Parkinson's disease	100 mg twice daily
Amantadine when given in combination with levodopa	Initiate with 100 mg daily
Drug-induced extrapyramidal reactions	100 mg twice daily

- *Central nervous system*: Hyperreflexia, convulsions, extrapyramidal signs (torsion spasms, dystonic posturing), motor restlessness, depressed level of consciousness, dysphagia, confusion, dilated pupils, delirium, disorientation, myoclonus, aggression/hostility, visual hallucinations, and can even lead to coma.
- *Respiratory system*: Hyperventilation, respiratory distress, pulmonary edema, and acute respiratory distress.
- *Cardiovascular system*: Hypertension, sinus tachycardia, and arrhythmia. Additionally, cardiac arrest and sudden cardiac death are also reported.

Management of Overdosage

- Induction of vomiting and/or gastric aspiration and lavage if the patient is conscious should be undertaken.[3]
- Acidification of the urine should be done, which causes excretion of amantadine in the urine.[3]
- Monitor blood pressure, heart rate, electrocardiogram (ECG), respiration, body temperature, and treat for possible hypotension and cardiac arrhythmias, as necessary.[3]
- Slow administration of intravenous (IV) physostigmine, which effectively controls central nervous system manifestations.[2]

ADVERSE EFFECTS

Amantadine has a very low side effect profile, which at the recommended dosage ranges between 5 and 10% (**Table 2**).[1] Some of the adverse events (AEs) include confusion, blurred vision, visual hallucinations, constipation, and foot edema. Behavioral symptoms characteristic of impulse control disorders including hypersexuality, pathological gambling, and compulsive spending/eating are also reported. Other AEs include nausea, dry mouth, livedo reticularis, somnolence, dizziness, anxiety, and depression.[4]

TABLE 2: Adverse effects of amantadine.[3]

Nervous system disorders

Uncommon	Dizziness, headache, lethargy, ataxia, and dysarthria
Rare	Tremor, dyskinesia, and convulsion
Very rare	Neuroleptic malignant syndrome (NMS)-like symptoms

Psychiatric disorders

Uncommon	Depression, anxiety, elevated mood, and agitation
Rare	Confusion state, disorientation, and psychotic disorder

Eye disorders

Uncommon	Blurring of vision
Rare	• Corneal lesions—punctate subepithelial and other corneal opacities • Corneal epithelial degradation, presenting as visual blurring, which is reversible on reducing amantadine

Cardiac disorders

Uncommon	Palpitations
Very rare	Cardiac failure

Vascular disorder

Uncommon	Orthostatic hypotension

Blood and lymphatic system disorder

Very rare	Leukopenia

Gastrointestinal disorders

Uncommon	Dry mouth, nausea, vomiting, and constipation
Rare	Diarrhea

Continued

Continued

Metabolism and nutrition disorder	
Uncommon	Decreased appetite
Other side effect	
Common	Peripheral edema

The acute AEs of amantadine appear within the first 2 days of treatment and promptly disappear within 24–48 hours after treatment discontinuation.[3] Chronic adverse effects may come slowly which are also dose dependent.

MONITORING

While administering amantadine, patient's renal function, blood pressure, and mental status may be monitored. Also, liver enzymes in patients with liver disease should be checked regularly as an irreversible elevation in transaminases has been reported.[4] Following parameters or symptoms should be watched for:

- *Renal function*: Any elevation in creatinine and blood urea nitrogen (BUN) or reduction in glomerular filtration rate (GFR)
- *Mental status*: Ask regarding any history of hallucinations, delusions, depression, and suicidal ideations
- *Blood pressure*: Look for orthostatic hypotension
- *Liver function test (LFT)*: Any increase in aspartate aminotransferase (AST) and alanine aminotransferase (ALT)

Additionally, an association between Parkinson's disease and the incidence of melanoma has been seen; therefore, it is essential to have periodic skin examinations.[4]

CONTRAINDICATIONS

Patients with hypersensitivity to drugs should be monitored while consuming amantadine.

Extended-release dosage form of amantadine is contraindicated in patients with end-stage renal disease as amantadine undergoes renal excretion.[4]

Amantadine should be avoided in patients with severe dopa-agonist-induced psychosis.

The drug is not advisable to pregnant women as it has shown to have teratogenic potential in animal studies. It is important to weigh the benefit to risk ratio while prescribing amantadine to breastfeeding mothers as it may risk infants.[4]

DRUG–DRUG INTERACTIONS

- When administering amantadine with central nervous stimulants, careful monitoring is recommended.[2]
- When taking amantadine with other CNS stimulants, it is important to monitor the patient.[2]
- Anticholinergic drugs may increase the anticholinergic side effects of amantadine.[2]
- Elderly patients with Parkinson's disease, coadministration of thioridazine could worsen tremor.[2]
- In a 61-year-old man receiving amantadine, 100 mg TID for Parkinson's disease experienced high drug plasma level when coadministered with triamterene/hydrochlorothiazide.[2]
- Reduction in renal clearance of amantadine by 30% is observed with coadministered with quinine or quinidine.[2]

SUMMARY

- Standard dose of amantadine is 100 mg twice daily when used alone with onset of action within 48 hours.
- When used with levodopa, amantadine is kept at a constant 100 mg daily or twice daily dosage while the dose of levodopa is gradually increased.
- Occasionally, patients whose responses are not optimal with amantadine 200 mg daily may benefit from an increase up to 300–400 mg daily in divided doses.

- Amantadine overdosage could result in cardiac, respiratory, renal, or central nervous system toxicity.
- Amantadine has a very low side effect profile, which at the recommended dosage ranges between 5 and 10% and includes nausea, dizziness (lightheadedness), and insomnia.
- While administering amantadine, patient monitoring for renal function, blood pressure, and mental status should be considered.

REFERENCES

1. Ciplamed. (2019). Amantrel capsules. [online] Available from https://www.ciplamed.com/content/amantrel-capsules. [Last accessed June, 2021].
2. Chang C, Ramphul K. Amantadine. Treasure Island: StatPearls Publishing; 2021.
3. Novartis. (2019). Symmetrel®: antiparkinsonian agent and anti-influenzal virostatic. [online] Available from https://www.novartis.com.sg/sites/www.novartis.com.sg/files/product-info/Symmetrel-Apr%202019.SIN-Approved28Jun19.pdf. [Last accessed June, 2021].
4. RxList. (2019). Symmetrel. [online] Available from https://www.rxlist.com/symmetrel-drug.htm#overdosage. [Last accessed June, 2020].

Index

Page numbers followed by f refer to figure, fc refer to flowchart, and t refer to table.

A

Akinesia 3
Alanine aminotransferase 46
Amantadine 16, 17, 19, 20, 21f, 22, 23, 25, 27-30, 32t, 34-39, 42, 44, 47, 48
   adverse effects of 42, 45t
   clearance of 23, 25t
   concentrations 25
   dosage 42, 43t
   dose of 42
   duration of 33
   effectiveness 34
   efficacy of 28
   exhibits 38
   general pharmacodynamics of 20
   mechanism of action of 20
   overdosage of 43
   pharmacokinetic properties of 24t
   safety of 28, 29
   structure of 20f
   therapy 35t, 36t
   treatment 34
   use of 37
Anticholinergics 16
Antidyskinetic effects 28
Antiparkinsonian drugs 42
Antiviral agent 37
Ataxia, management of 38

B

Blood 45
   pressure 46, 48
Blurred vision 44
Bradykinesia 3, 35, 36
Brain bank criteria 11

C

Cardiac disorders 45
Cardiovascular system 44
Central nervous system 44
Concomitant therapy, dosage for 42
Constipation 44
Corticostriatal tract 22f

D

Degenerative cerebellar ataxias 38
Dementia 6
Dizziness 48
Dopamine agonist 28
Dopaminergic
   medications 16
   pathway 38
   system 20
Drug–drug interactions 42, 47
Dyskinesia 33
   developed 29
   risk of 28
   levodopa-induced 17, 28

Index

E

End-stage renal disease 47
Erectile dysfunction 7
Extrapyramidal reactions, dosage for drug-induced 43

F

Freezing of gait 31
    efficacy of amantadine in 31
    questionnaire 33fc
    response 32t

G

Gait questionnaire score 33f
Gastric aspiration 44
Gastrointestinal disorders 45
Glutamatergic system 21

H

Hypokinesia 3
Hypophonia 4

I

Immunomodulation 21
Inspiratory respiratory dysfunction 14

L

Levodopa 13, 28
    treatment 20
Levodopa-induced dyskinesia, treatment of 29
Lewy body
    break staging of 11t
    deposition, staging of 11
Liver function test 46
Lymphatic system disorder 45

M

Mental status 46, 48
Metabolism 25, 46
Motor symptoms 4fc
Movement Disorder Society 13, 30
Multiple system atrophy 33fc, 34, 36

N

Nervous system disorders 45
Neurodegenerative movement disorder 1
Nigrostriatal nerve terminal 22f
N-methyl-d-aspartate 21f
Nonmotor symptoms 5, 5fc, 6, 7t
Noradrenergic pathway 38
Noradrenergic system 21
Nutrition disorder 46

O

Overdosage, management of 44
Oxidative stress 10

P

Parkinson's disease 1, 4fc, 5fc, 8, 10, 17, 21, 28, 33fc, 43, 46, 47
    advanced 7
    clinical signs and symptoms of 1
    diagnosis 10, 11, 14fc
    dosage for 42
    drug therapy 6
    early 28
    epidemiology of 1
    estimated prevalence of 2f
    idiopathic 23
    management of 15, 16t

pathophysiology 10
postural reflex impairment in 31
premotor 7t
risk factors of 3
role of amantadine in 19
severe 19, 33
supportive criteria for 12
symptoms 4f
Parkinson's hyperpyrexia syndrome 6
Parkinsonian syndrome bradykinesia, diagnosis of 12
Parkinsonism 35, 36
  signs of 3
  treatment of 22
Periodic skin examinations 46
Placebo arm 39
Plasma
  acetylamantadine 25
  amantadine concentration 30
  concentrations 26
  proteins 23
Postural instability 5
Potent neurotoxins 10
Presynaptic dopaminergic system 13
Primary progressive freezing gait 33fc
Progressive supranuclear palsy 33fc, 34, 35

Psychiatric
  disorders 45
  symptoms 8

Q

Quinidine 47
Quinine 47

R

Renal function 46
Respiratory system 44
Resting tremor 36
Rigidity 5

T

Thioridazine 47
Traumatic brain injury 38
  management of 38
Tremor 5

U

Unified dyskinesia rating scale 30

V

Visual hallucinations 44
Vomiting 44

EU GSPR Authorised Reprsentative
Logos Europe, 9 rue Nicolas Poussin
1700, La Rochelle, France
Phone: +33 (0) 6 67 93 73 78
E-mail: contact@logoseurope.eu

www.ingramcontent.com/pod-product-compliance
Ingram Content Group UK Ltd.
Pitfield, Milton Keynes, MK11 3LW, UK
UKHW021827140426
5217IPUK00016B/1230